Joana Perotta Titon

Meridian Theory, Vital Substances, Zang Fu and Five Elements

Joana Perotta Titon

Meridian Theory, Vital Substances, Zang Fu and Five Elements

Course Conclusion Work

ScienciaScripts

Imprint
Any brand names and product names mentioned in this book are subject to trademark, brand or patent protection and are trademarks or registered trademarks of their respective holders. The use of brand names, product names, common names, trade names, product descriptions etc. even without a particular marking in this work is in no way to be construed to mean that such names may be regarded as unrestricted in respect of trademark and brand protection legislation and could thus be used by anyone.

Cover image: www.ingimage.com

This book is a translation from the original published under ISBN 978-613-9-68159-4.

Publisher:
Sciencia Scripts
is a trademark of
Dodo Books Indian Ocean Ltd. and OmniScriptum S.R.L publishing group

120 High Road, East Finchley, London, N2 9ED, United Kingdom
Str. Armeneasca 28/1, office 1, Chisinau MD-2012, Republic of Moldova, Europe
Printed at: see last page
ISBN: 978-620-8-19456-7

index:

1. meridian theory

The oldest reference to Meridian Theory is in the book Hwang Ti Nei Jing. It contains precise descriptions of its principles.

The meridians (*Tin* or *Jing*) were described from regions of the human body which, after acupuncture, generated a sensation of heat and paresthesia that followed similar directions. They connect the organs and viscera to the skin, muscles, tendons, bones and other tissues. The analogous points are distributed longitudinally. The connection of points transversely gave rise to the so-called *Lo* or *Luo* (communications).

Twelve ordinary meridians have been established and are directly related to organs and viscera in the body. From them there are branches that run through cavities in the body, the distinct or divergent meridians. The meridians that connect the ordinary meridians are fifteen in number and are called *Lo-Mai* (connected meridians). There are two other types of meridians that make connections: superficial collaterals and minimal collaterals. There are twelve muscle-tendon meridians and twelve superficial meridians (on the trunk and limbs).

The ordinary meridians are coupled in pairs, where a superficial meridian is always coupled to a deep one. The Yin meridians belong to the organs and their Lo correspondent to the viscera, while the Yang meridians belong to the viscera and their Lo correspondent to the organs. The superficial meridians are linked by Lo connections. At the ends of the fingers of the limbs are the connections between the superficial and deep meridians.

The five elements have the following relationship with the meridians: a) Wood: liver - superficial; gall bladder - deep b) Fire: heart and pericardium - superficial; small intestine and triple heater - deep

c)   Earth: spleen-pancreas - superficial; stomach - deep

d)   Metal: lung - superficial; large intestine - deep

e) Water: kidney - superficial; bladder - deep

The meridians have the function of ensuring good circulation of the body's trophic-physiological factors, which are: Chi - energy, Xue - blood, Ying - nutrition (intravascular nutritional factor), Wei - defense (extravascular defensive factor). With the function of connecting the organs and viscera and the four extremities externally, the meridians and collaterals carry Qi and Xue to moisten and nourish the body, making the balance between inside and outside, upper and lower, anterior and posterior. They are responsible for maintaining physiological functions, regulating the balance between Yin and Yang. They protect the body from external pathogenic factors that try to invade through the skin. The protective function is performed by the Wei Qi (defense Qi), which fills the collaterals and regulates the opening and closing of the sweat pores, moistening and warming the skin and muscles.

Based on the theory of Yin and Yang, Yang meridians of the hand, Yang meridians of the leg, Yin meridians of the hand and Yin meridians of the leg were established. There is a relationship between the yin and yang meridians of the hands and feet and their effects. They are classified from the most Yin to the most Yang as follows:

a) Tai Yin - Major Yin: lung meridian (hand Yin) and spleen-pancreas meridian (leg Yin);

b) Jue Yin - Yin of transfer: meridian of the pericardium (Yin of the hand) and the liver (Yin of the leg);

c) Shao Yin - Minor Yin: meridian of the heart (hand Yin) and kidney (leg Yin);

d) Yang Ming - combination of Yang: meridian of the large intestine (Yang of the hand) and the stomach (Yang of the leg);

e) Shao Yang - Lesser Yang: meridian of the triple heater (Yang of the hand) and the gallbladder (Yang of the leg);

f) Tai Yang - Greater Yang: meridian of the small intestine (Yang of the hand)

and the bladder (yang of the leg).

The diagram below represents the six levels described:

ID <u>Tai Yang</u> B

TA <u>Shao Yang</u> VB

IG <u>Yang Ming</u> E

P <u>Tai Yin</u> BP

PC <u>Jue Yin</u> F

C <u>Shao Yin</u> R

It is a flow between the ordinary meridians, where there is an interconnection between them. The flow of Qi and Xue occurs as follows:

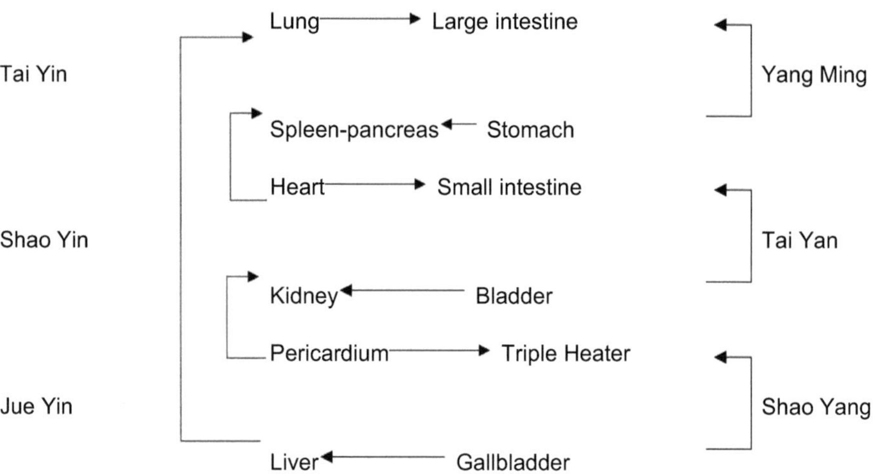

There are also countless other connections between the meridians, amounting to more than a hundred meridians that can be used in the patient's therapy.

The main meridians follow paths in the body according to their Yin or Yang characteristics. The three Yin meridians of the hand start in the chest and abdomen and run towards the hand. The three Yang meridians of the hand run from the hand to the head. The three Yang meridians of the foot start at the head and end at the feet. The three Yin meridians of the foot leave from the

4

feet and go towards the abdomen and chest.

On the palmar side of the upper limbs are three Yin meridians: lung, pericardium and heart. On the dorsal side, there are three Yang meridians: the large intestine, the triple heater and the small intestine. On the lower limbs, there are three Yin meridians on the medial side of the femur and tibia bones: spleen-pancreas, liver and kidneys; and three Yang meridians on the lateral and dorsal edge of the leg: stomach, gallbladder and bladder.

The head is the region where the Yang meridians of the upper limbs arrive and from where the meridians of the lower limbs depart. The Yang Ming are distributed on the face, the Shao Yang on the side of the head, the Tai Yang of the hand in the temporal region and of the leg in the parietal region.

In the torso, the meridians are distributed as follows: Yang Ming and Tai Yang on the ventral side, Shao Yang and Jue Yin on the lateral side. The Shao Yin meridians run along the center line of the ventral part of the torso, and the Tai Yin meridians run along the back of the torso.

The three Yin meridians from the leg ascend to the torso, from where they flow into the arms. The meridians are connected both superficially and deeply, making them a closed and complete system. When the body is affected by a pathogenic factor, it can unbalance the energy flow of a particular meridian. If this imbalance remains, it leads to syndromes related to the corresponding organs and viscera. Depending on the syndrome caused, it is possible to stimulate the acupuncture points responsible for balancing and maintaining the harmonious energy flow and then resolve the illness.

When a pathological condition occurs, the meridians and collaterals can transmit disease and reflect local and systemic signs and symptoms. Initially, the manifestations occur in the meridians and collaterals, and if they are not combated, they internalize into the organs and viscera.

Acupuncture helps treat these pathological conditions by stimulating the regulation of the deficiency or excess present in the affected meridian. The sensation of the "arrival of Qi" is essential for this treatment to be effective, a sensation characterized by pain, numbness, heaviness and distension at the punctured point.

Regular Meridians

Each main meridian contains its own points distributed in a fixed way on the body surface. There is a Zang or a Fu to which this meridian belongs and there is an interior-exterior relationship of mutual connection.

a) Heart Meridian: Shao Yin of the hand:

C1 Ji Quan	C6 Yin Xi
C2 Qing Ling	C7 Shen MEn
C3 Shao Hai	C8 Shao Fu
C4 Ling Dao	C9 Shao Chong
C5 Tong Li	

b) Kidney Meridian: Shao Yin of the foot:

R1 Yong Quan	R15 Zhong Zhu
R2 Ran Gu	R16 Huang Shu
R3 Tai Xi	R17 Shang Qu
R4 Da Zhong	R18 Shu Guan
R5 Shui Quan	R19 Yin Du
R6 Zhao Hai	R20 Fu Tong Gu
R7 Fu Liu	R21 You Men
R8 Jiao Xin	R22 Bu Lang
R8 Zhu Bin	R23 Sheng Feng
R10 Yin Gu	R24 Ling Xu
R11 Heng Gu	R25 Shen Cang
R12 Da He	R26 Yu Zhong
R13 Qi Xue	R27 Shu Fu
R14 Si Man	

c) Pericardium meridian: Jue Yin of the hand:

PC1 Tian Chi	PC6 Nei Guan
PC2 Tian Quan	PC7 Da Ling
PC3 Qu Ze	PC8 Lao Gang
PC4 Xi Men	PC9 Zhang Chang
PC5 Jian Xi	

d) Liver Meridian: Jue Yin of the foot:

F1 Da Dun	F8 Qu Quan
F2 Xing Jian	F9 Yin Bao
F3 Tai Chong	F10 Zu Wu Li
F4 Zhong Feng	F11 Yin Lian

F5 Li Gou	F12 Ji Mai
F6 Zhong Du	F13 Zhang Men
F7 Xi Guan	F14 Qi Men

e) Lung Meridian: Tai Yin of the hand:

P1 Zhang Fu	P7 Lie Que
P2 Yu Men	P8 Jing Qu
P3 Tian Fu	P9 Tai Yuan
P4 Xia Bai	P10 Yu Ji
P5 Chi Ze	P11 Shao Shang
P6 Kong Zui	

f) Spleen-Pancreas Meridian: Tai Yin of the foot:

BP1 Yin Bai	BP12 Chong Men
BP2 Da Du	BP 13 Fu She
BP3 Tai Bai	BP14 Fu Jie
BP4 Gong Sun	BP15 Da Heng
BP5 Shang Qiu	BP16 Fu Ai
BP6 San Yin Jiao	BP17 Shi Dou
BP7 Lou Gu	BP18 Tian Xi
BP8 Di Ji	BP19 Xiong Xiang
BP9 Yin Ling Quan	BP20 Zhou Rong
BP10 Xue Hai	BP21 Da Bao
BP11 Ji Men	

g) Large Intestine Meridian: Yang Ming of the hand:

IG1 Shang Yang	IG5 Yang Xi
IG2 Er Jian	IG6 Pian Li
IG 3 San Jian	IG7 Wen Liu
IG4 He Gu	IG8 Xai Lian
IG9 Shang Lian IG10 Shou	IG15 Jian Yu
San Li IG11 Qu Chi IG12	IG16 Ju Gu
Zhou Liao	IG17 Tian Ding
IG13 Shou Wu Li	IG18 Fu Tu
IG14 Bi No	IG19 Kou He Liao
	IG20 Ying Xiang

h) Stomach Meridian: Yang Ming of the foot:

E1 Cheng Qi	E24 Hua Rou Men
E2 Si Bai	E25 Tian Shu
E3 Ju Liao	E26 Wai Ling
E4 Di Cang	Ju's E27
E5 Da Yang	E28 Shui Dao
E6 Jia Che	E29 Gui Lai
E7 Xia Guan	E30 Qi Chong
E8 Tou Wei	E31 Bi Guan
E9 Ren Ying	E32 Fu Tu
E10 Shui Tu	E33 Yin Shi
E11 Qi She	E34 Liang Qiu

E12 Que Pen
E13 Qi Hu
E14 Ku Fang
E15 Wu Yi
E16 TYing Chuang
E17 Ru Zhong
E18 Ru Gen
E19 Bu Rong
E20 Cheng Man
E21 Liang Men
E22 Guan Men
E23 Tai Ti
E35 Du Bi
E36 Zu San Li
E37 Shang Ju Xu
E38 Tiao Kou
E39 Xia Ju Xu
E40 Feng Long
E41 Jie Xi
E42 Chong Yanh
E43 Xian Gu
E44 Nei Ting
E45 Li Dui

i) San Jiao Meridian (Triple Heater): Shao Yang da hand:

TA1 Guan Chong
TA2 Ye Men
TA3 Zhang Zhu
TA4 Yang Chi
TA5 Wai Guan
TA6 Zhi Gou
TA7 Hui Zhong
TA8 San Yang Luo
TA9 Si Du
TA10 Tian Jing
TA11 Qing Leng Yuan
TA12 Xiao Luo
TA13 Nao Shi
TA14 Jiao Liao
TA15 Tian Liao
TA16 Tian You
TA17 Yi Feng
TA18 Chi Mai
TA19 Lu Xi
TA20 Jiao Sun
TA21 Er Men
TA22 Er He Liao
TA23 Si Zhu Kong

j) Gallbladder Meridian: Shao Yang of the foot:

VB1 Tong Zi Liao
VB2 Ting Hui
VB3 Shang Guan
VB4 Han Yan
VB5 Xuan Lu
VB6 Xuan Li
VB7 Qu Bin
VB8 Suai Gu
VB9 Tian Chong
VB10 Fu Bai
VB11 Tou Qiao Yin
VB12 Wan Gu
VB13 Well Shen
VB14 Yang Bai
VB15 Tou Lin Qi
VB16 Mu Chuang
VB17 Zheng Ying
VB18 Cheng Ling
VB23 Zhe Jin
VB24 Ri Yue
VB25 Jing Men
VB26 Dai Mai
VB27 Wu Shu
VB28 Wei Dao
VB29 Ju Liao
VB30 Huan Tiao
VB31 Feng Shi
VB32 Zhong Du
VB33 Xi Yang Guan
VB34 Yang Ling Quan
VB35 Yang Jiao
VB36 Qai Qiu
VB37 Guang Ming
VB38 Yang Fu
VB39 Xuan Zhong
VB40 Qiu Xu

VB19 No Kong
VB20 Feng Chi
VB21 Jian Jing
VB22 Yuan Ye
VB41 Zu Lin Qi
VB42 Di Wu Hui
VB43 Xia Xi
VB44 Zu Qiao Yin

k) Small Intestine Meridian: Tai Yang of the hand:

ID1 Shao Ze
ID2 Qian Gu
ID3 Hou Xi
ID4 Wan Gu
ID5 Yang Gu
ID6 Yang Lao
ID7 Zhi Zheng
ID8 Xiao Hai
ID9 Jian Zhen
ID10 Nao Shu
ID11 Tian Zong
ID12 Bing Feng
ID13 Qu Yuan
ID14 Jian Wai Shu
ID15 Jian Zhong Shu
ID16 Tian Chuang
ID17 Tian Rong
ID18 Quan Liao
ID19 Ting Gong

l) Bladder Meridian: Tai Yang of the foot:

B1 Jing Ming
B2 Zan Zhu
B3 Mei Chong
B4 Qu Chai
B5 Wu Chu
B6 Cheng Guang
B7 Tong Tian
B8 Luo Que
B9 Yu Zhen
B10 Tian Zhu
B11 Da Zhu
B12 Feng Men
B13 Fei Shu
B14 Jue Yin Shu
B15 Xin Shu
B16 Du Shu
B17 Ge Shu
B18 Gan Shu
B19 Dan Shu
B20 Pi Shu
B21 Wei Shu
B22 San Jiao Shu
B23 Shen Shu
B24 Qi Hai Shu
B25 Da Chang Shu
B26 Guan Yuan Shu
B27 Xiao Chang Shu
B28 Pang Guang Shu
B29 Zhong Lu Shu
B30 Bai Huan Shu
B31 Shang Liao
B37 Yin Men
B38 Fu Xi
B39 Wei Yang
B40 Wei Zhong
B41 Fu Fen
B42 Po Hu
B43 Gao Huang
B44 Shen Tang
B45 Yi Xi
B46 Ge Guan
B47 Hun Men
B48 Yang Gang
B49 Yi She
B50 Wei Cang
B51 Huang Men
B52 Zi Shi
B53 Bao Huang
B54 Zhi Bian
B55 He Yang
B56 Cheng Jin
B57 Cheng Shan
B58 Fei Yang
B59 Fu Yang
B60 Kun Lun
B61 Pu Shen
B62 Shen Mai
B63 Jin Men

B32 Ci Liao	B64 Jing Gu
B33 Zhang Liao	B65 Shu Gu
B34 Xia Liao	B66 Zu Tong Gu
B35 Hui Yang	B67 Zhi Yin
B36 Cheng Fu	

There is a normal variation in the quantity of Qi and Xue in the twelve meridians under physiological conditions. These quantities are in relative balance through inner-external interrelationships. While the Tai Yang meridian has a lot of Xue and less Qi, its related Shao Yin meridian has the opposite. The Shao Yang meridian has less Xue and a lot of Qi, and its related Jue Yin meridian has the opposite. The Yang Ming meridian, on the other hand, has a unique characteristic of a lot of Qi and Xue, because it is indispensable from birth and is the source of growth and transformation. Its related meridian, Tai Yin, has a lot of Qi and less Xue. This variation in Qi and Xue serves as the basis for treatment, with tonification and sedation of acupuncture points.

Meridians Mai Extras

The Mai Extra meridians are eight in total and largely connect the regular, divergent and collateral meridians to each other. They control and regulate the Qi and Xue of the whole body. They drain and store them when they are in excess and supply Qi and Xue when they are deficient.

Some of the characteristics of these eight meridians differ from the main meridians. They don't penetrate or connect with the Zang Fu directly, nor do they have an interior-exterior relationship. Only two meridians, Du Mai and Ren, have their own points, the other six share points with the regular meridians. They strengthen the associations between the regular meridians and act as regulators and stores for the Qi of these meridians. Three of these meridians originate in the uterus and emerge in the perineum: Du Mai, Ren Mai and Chong Mai. They are called "three branches from the same origin".

a)   Du Mai: runs along the midline of the back and ascends to the head and face. It is called the "sea of Yang meridians" because it governs and controls the Yang meridians and during its course it crosses the Yang meridians of the hand and foot at point DM14, and the Yang Wei Mai at points DM15 and DM16. It is closely related to the brain, spinal cord and kidney.

DM1 Chang Qiang	DM15 Ya Men
DM2 Yao Shu	DM16 Feng Fu
DM3 Yao Yang Guan	DM17 Nao Hu
DM4 Ming Men	DM18 Qiang Jian
DM5 Xuan Shu	DM19 Hou Ding
DM6 Ji Zhong	DM20 Bai Hui
DM7 Zhong Shu	DM21 Qian Ding
DM8 Jin Suo	DM22 Xin Hui
DM9 Zhi Yang	DM 23 Shang Xing
DM10 Ling Tai	DM24 Shen Ting
DM11 Shen Dao	DM25 Su Liao
DM12 Shen Zhu	DM26 Shui Gou
DM13 Tao Dao	DM27 Dui Duan
DM14 Da Zhui	DM28 Yin Jiao

b)   Ren Mai: runs along the midline of the abdomen, crosses the Yin meridians of the hand and foot at points RM3 and RM4 and crosses the Yin Wei Mai at points RM22 and RM23, making it responsible for all the Yin meridians. It is called the "sea of Yin meridians", since Xue (Yin) is related to pregnancy, childbirth, menstruation and vaginal discharge. It starts in the uterus and helps with the functions of nourishment, conception, pregnancy and the growth of the fetus.

RM1 Hui Yin	RM13 Shang Wan
RM2 Qu Gu	RM14 Ju Que
RM3 Zhong Ji	RM15 Jiu Wei
RM4 Guan Yuan	RM16 Zhong Ting
RM5 Shi Men	RM17 Dan Zhong
RM6 Qi Hai	RM18 Yu Tang
RM7 Yin Jiao	RM19 Zi Gong
RM8 Shen Que	RM20 Hua Gai
RM9 Shui Fen	RM21 Xuan Ji
RM10 Xia Wan	RM22 Tian Tu
RM11 Jian Li	RM23 Lian Quan
RM12 Zhong Wan	RM24 Cheng Jiang

c)   Chong Mai: controls the Qi and Xue of all the meridians, then called the "sea of the twelve regular meridians" and the "sea of Xue". It originates in the uterus and is related to menstruation. It meets the Shao Yin meridian of the foot and the Yang Ming meridian of the hand.

RM1 Hui Yin	RM7 Yin Jiao
E30 Qi Chong	R16 Huang Shu
R11 Heng Gu	R17 Shang Qu
R12 Da He	R18 Shu Guan
R13 Qi Xue	R19 Yin Du
R14 Si Man	R20 Fu Tong Gu
R15 Zhong Zhu	R21 You Men

d)   Dai Mai: originates in the hypochondrium and passes around the waist, connecting all the vertical meridians.

VB26 Dai Mai

VB27 Wu Shu

VB28 Wei Dao

e)   Yin Wei Mai and Yang Wei Mai: connect and interconnect the Yin and Yang meridians of the entire body, respectively.

The Yin Wei Mai joins the Ren Mai at points RM22 and RM23. The Yang Wei Mai joins the Du Mai at DM 15 and

DM16.
- Yin Wei Mai:

RM22 Tian Tu	BP15 Da Heng
RM23 Lian Quan	BP13 Fu She
F14 Qi Mei	R9 Zhu Bin
BP16 Fu Ai	

- Yang Wei Mai:

VB14 Yang Bai	VB20 Feng Chi
VB13 Well Shen	TA15 Tian Liao
VB15 Tou Lin Qi	VB21 Jian Jing
VB17 Zheng Yin	ID10 Nao Shu
VB19 No Kong	VB25 Yang Jiao
DM15 Ya Men	B63 Jin Men
DM16 Feng Fu	

f)   Yin Qiao Mai and Yang Qiao Mai: start below the inner and outer malleolus respectively. Both are located in the medial corner of the eye and can nourish the eyes. They are also responsible for opening and closing the eyes. Their common function is to move the lower limbs.

- Yin Qiao Mai
B1 Jing Ming
R8 Jiao Xin
- Yang Qiao Mai
B1 Jing Ming
E1 Cheng Qi
E3 Ju Liao
E4 Di Cang
IG16 Ju Gu
ID10 Nao Shu

R2 Ran Gu
R6 Zhao Hai

IG15 Jian Yu
VB29 Ju Liao
B59 Fu Yang
B61 Pu Shen
B62 Shen Mai

Diverging Meridians

These are important branches that separate from the twelve regular meridians and run towards the chest, abdomen and head, from the four limbs. They connect the related inner and outer meridians and strengthen the association between the meridians and the Zang-Fu. They are an extension of the Zang-Fu meridians and extend the treatment indications of the regular meridians because they run through deep regions of the body.

The behavior of these twelve divergent meridians boils down to drifting, entering, emerging and uniting.

Divergent Meridian from the Bladder Meridian - Tai Yang of the foot: derives from the popliteal fossa, runs up to 5 cun below the sacrum, goes around the anal region, connects with the bladder and distributes itself in the kidney. It follows the spine, distributes itself in the heart region and emerges in the neck, where it joins the Bladder meridian.

Divergent Meridian of the Kidney Meridian - Shao Yin of the foot: diverges from the regular meridian in the popliteal fossa, crosses the divergent meridian of the bladder in the thigh, connects to the kidney, crosses the Dai Mai at the level of the seventh thoracic vertebra, ascends to the root of the tongue and emerges at the nape of the neck to connect to the meridian of the Bladder, Tai Yang of the foot.

Divergent Meridian of the Large Intestine Meridian - Yang Ming of the hand: separates from the stomach meridian in the thigh, penetrates the abdomen, connects with the stomach, disperses in the spleen, ascends through the heart, runs along the esophagus until it reaches the mouth. It continues upwards next to the nose and connects with the eye before joining the meridian of the stomach, Yang Ming of the foot.

Divergent meridian of the spleen-pancreas meridian - Tai Yin of the foot: derives from the spleen-pancreas meridian in the thigh, converges with the divergent meridian of the stomach, continues upwards to the throat and enters the tongue.

Divergent Meridian of the Gallbladder Meridian - Shao Yang of the foot: derives from the regular meridian in the thigh, crosses the hip joint, enters the lower abdomen in the pelvic region, converges with the divergent meridian of the liver, passes between the ribs, connects to the gallbladder, distributes through the liver, continues upwards through the heart and esophagus, disperses on the face, connects with the eye and joins the meridian of the gallbladder, Shao Yang of the foot, in the outer corner of the foot.

Divergent Meridian from the Liver Meridian - Jue Yin of the foot: separates from the regular meridian on the back of the foot, goes to the pubic region, converges with the gallbladder meridian, Shao Yang of the foot.

Divergent Meridian of the Small Intestine Meridian - Tai Yang of the hand: separates from the regular meridian at the shoulder joint, enters the armpit, crosses the heart, runs down the bar to the abdomen, where it connects with the small intestine meridian.

Meridian Divergent from the Heart Meridian - Shao Yin of the hand: derives from the regular meridian in the axillary fossa, penetrates the chest, connects with the heart, ascends through the throat, emerges on the face, joins with the Small Intestine meridian in the inner corner of the eye.

Divergent Meridian of the Large Intestine Meridian - Yang Ming of the hand: separates from the regular meridian in the hand, goes upwards along the arm and shoulder and into the chest. One branch diverges at the top of the shoulder and enters the spine at the nape of the neck, goes downwards and joins the large intestine and lung. Another branch ascends from the shoulder along the throat, emerges in the supraclavicular fossa, then rejoins the Large Intestine meridian.

Divergent Meridian from the Lung Meridian - Tai Yin of the hand: derives from the lung meridian in the armpit, continues

anteriorly to the path of the pericardium meridian inside the thorax, connects with the lung, disperses in the large intestine. A branch goes upwards from the lung and emerges at the clavicle, ascends along the throat and converges with the meridian of the large intestine.

Divergent Meridian from the Triple Heater Meridian - Shao Yang of the hand: separates from the regular meridian at the vertex, descends into the supraclavicular fossa and crosses the Upper, Middle and Lower Heater (Jiao), then disperses into the thorax.

Meridian Divergent from the Pericardium Meridian - Jue Yin of the hand: originates in the pericardium meridian 3 cun below the armpit, enters the chest and communicates with the Triple Heater. A branch ascends through the throat, emerges behind the ear and converges with the Triple Heater meridian.

Tendinomuscular Meridians

These meridians connect to the tendons, muscles and tissues. They are nourished and supplied by their corresponding regular meridians. They start at the distal point of the extremities and run through the prominence of the muscles to the large joints or the genital regions.

Their role is to integrate the body so that the structures work synergistically, maintaining the normal movements of the muscles and joints. They have no connection with the Zang-Fu, although some meridians go deeper.

Based on the area affected, the form of treatment is determined, starting with the painful points, also called Ah-Shi, according to the tendon-muscle meridian affected.

The meridians are described below:

a)   Tai Yang of the foot: distributes through the fifth toe of the foot, passes through the external malleolus, heel, knee, popliteal fossa, nape, paraspinal region, shoulders, supraclavicular fossa, nape of the neck, root of the tongue, occipital bone, head, nose, supraorbital region, paranasal region and mastoid process.

b)   Shao Yang of the foot: distributed over the fourth toe, external malleolus, lateral aspect of the knee, fibula, thigh, point E32, nape, hypochondria, anterior axillary region, costal region, supraclavicular fossa, region posterior to the ear, angle of the forehead, vertex, mandible, nose, external corner of the eyelid.

c)   Yang Ming of the foot: distributed over the third toe, dorsum of the foot, lateral aspect of the knee, tibia, fibula, thigh, hip joint, hypochondria, spine, genital organs, sternum, abdomen, supraclavicular fossa, neck, mouth, side of the nose, supranasal region, infraorbital region, region anterior to the ear.

d)   Tai Yin of the foot: distributed over the medial surface of the hallux, internal malleolus, lower tibia, medial surface of the thigh, point B31, external genital organ, abdomen, navel, inner abdomen, hypochondrium, thoracic cavity, spine.

e)   Shao Yin of the foot: distributed on the inside of the fifth toe, below the internal malleolus, the lower part of the tibia, the lateral aspect of the thigh, the external genital organ, the inside of the spine, the para-spinal muscles, the back of the neck, the occipital bone.

f)   Jue Yin of the foot: distributed over the hallux, anterior to the medial malleolus, calf, lower part of the tibia, medial aspect of the thigh, external genital organs.

g)   Tai Yang of the hand: distributed over the little finger, wrist, medial epicondyle of the humerus, armpit, scapula, neck, mastoid process, inner ear, supra-auricular region, mandible, outer corner of the eyelid, forehead.

h)   Shao Yang of the hand: distributed over the fourth finger, wrist, forearm, elbow, shoulder, side of the arm, neck, jaw, throat, base of the tongue, area before the ear, outer angle of the eye and forehead.

i)   Yang Ming of the hand: distributed over the index finger, wrist, side of the forearm, elbow, arm, shoulder, back, neck, angle of the jaw, maxilla, forehead and skull.

j)   Tai Yin of the hand: distributed over the thumb, forearm, elbow, upper arm, armpit, supraclavicular fossa, shoulder and chest.

k)   Shao Yin of the hand: distributed over the fifth finger, ulnar side of the wrist, forearm, inner region of the elbow, armpit, chest and umbilical scar.

l)   Jue Yin of the hand: distributed over the middle finger of the hand, palm of the hand, anterior surface of the forearm, elbow, ulnar surface of the arm, armpit, thorax and diaphragm.

Skin Regions

The skin regions follow the nomenclature of the six meridian levels and correspond to the twelve regular and collateral meridians. They are nourished by the Qi and Xue of their correlated and collateral meridians. External pathogenic factors can invade the interior of the body by affecting these regions. It also serves as a parameter for evaluating skin color and luster changes, hardened bumps or nodules under the skin, abnormal sensations in the skin and any other sign that can help in the diagnosis of diseases present in the meridians. Below is the distribution of the skin regions on the left side of the body:

Figure 1: Distribution of skin regions.

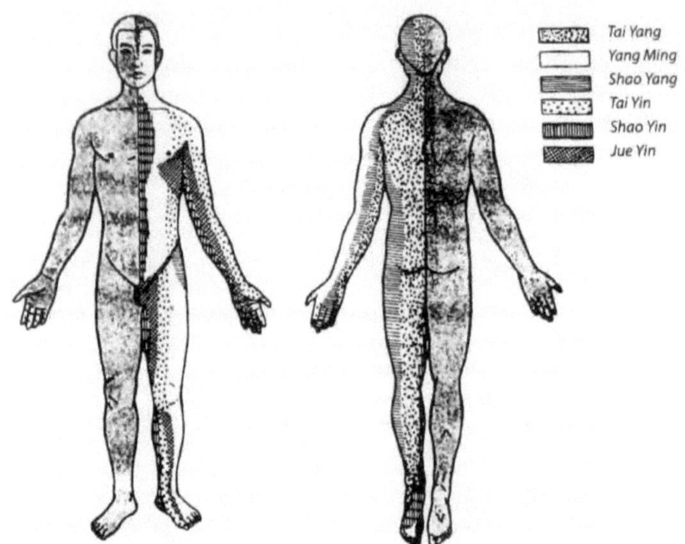

Source: Tratado contemporàneo de Acupuntura e Moxibustâo, Brazilian edition Hong Jin Pai, 2005

Collateral Meridians

The collateral meridians derive from the twelve regular meridians, there is also a large spleen collateral, a Du Mai and Ren Mai collateral, making a total of fifteen collateral meridians.

The collaterals of the regular meridians start at the Luo and go to their related inner-exterior meridians (the Yang go to the related inner-exterior Yin and vice versa).

Their main function is to strengthen the association between the inner and outer meridians through the Luo points. A very effective method of treatment is to combine the Yuan (Source) point with the Luo (Connection) point.

There are also other smaller collaterals. Those that pass through the surface of the skin are called Superficial Collaterals and the branches of the smaller collaterals are called Minimal Collaterals. Their function is also to transport Qi and Xue. It can be used with the method of bleeding these points to treat illnesses.

Below are the fifteen collaterals:

Name of collateral	Luo Points (Connection)
Tai Yin of the Hand	Lie Que (P7)
Jue Yin of the Hand	Nei Guan (PC6)
Shao Yin of the Hand	Tong Li (C5)
Yang Ming of the Hand	Pian Li (IG6)
Shao Yang of the Hand	Wai Guan (TA5)
Tai Yang of the Hand	Zhi Zheng (ID7)
Yang Ming of the Foot	Feng Long (E4O)
Shao Yang of the Foot	Guang Ming (VB37)
Tai Yang of the Foot	Fei Yang (B58)
Tai Yin of the Foot	Gong Sun (BP4)
Shao Yin of the Foot	Da Zhong (R4)
Jue Yin of the Foot	Li Gou (F5)
Ren Mai	Jiu Wei (RM15)
Du Mai	Chang Qiang (DM1)
Pi's Big Collateral	Da Bao (BP21)

2. Theory of Vital Substances

Vital substances represent Qi in various forms of materiality, from bodily fluids to the immaterial form Shen (Mind). The interaction of these substances results in the function of the body and mind. They are: Qi, Xen, Jing, Jin Ye and Shen.

IQ

Qi has a versatile nature, it varies from something rarefied and material to something dense and material, and can be referred to as an "energy". It manifests itself simultaneously on the physical and material levels, and has a constant state of flow in varying states of aggregation. Its functions are to transform, transport, maintain, rise, protect and heat.

a)   Yuan Qi (Original Qi): is the Essence in the form of Qi that begins between the two kidneys. It is the origin of Yuan Yin and Yuan Yang. It depends on the nourishment of the post-Celestial Essence. It is a dynamic driving force for all the organs, circulating through the channels. It is also the basis of the Kidney's Qi, relating to all the Kidney's functional activities. It aids the transformation of

Zong Qi into Zhen Qi. The Triple Heater is the driving force for the Original Qi to differentiate into its various forms in different places throughout the body and it is stored in the source points (Yuan). Yuan Qi facilitates the transformation of Gu into Xen in Xin.

b)   Gu Qi (Food Qi): Food enters the Stomach and with the help of the Spleen is transformed into Gu Qi. It rises from the Middle Heater to the chest and goes into the lungs. It combines with the air to form Zong Qi. It then goes to the Heart where it is transformed into Xen with the help of Kidney Qi and Original Qi.

c)   Zong Qi (Gathering, Ancestral or Thoracic Qi): comes from the interaction of Gu Qi with the air. It helps the Lung and Heart in their functions of controlling Qi, breathing, Xen and blood vessels. They send Qi to the limbs, especially the hands. It also accumulates in the throat and influences speech and strengthens the voice.

d)   Zhen Qi (True Qi): Zong Qi is transformed into Zhen Qi under the catalytic action of Yuan Qi. It also originates in the lungs. It exists in two forms: Ying Qi and Wei Qi.

e)   Ying Qi (Nutritive Qi): nourishes the internal organs and the whole organism, has an intimate relationship with Xuw and flows with it through the blood vessels and into the channels.

f)   Wei Qi (Defensive Qi): Flows in the outer layers of the body, has a Yang characteristic. Its function is to protect the body from external pathogenic factors such as wind, heat, cold and humidity. It partially warms, moisturizes and nourishes the skin and muscles, controls the opening and closing of pores (regulates sweating) and regulates body temperature. It is under the control of the Lung. Wei Qi circulates 50 times in 24 hours, 25 times during the day on the outside of the yang surface channels and 25 times at night in the yin organs.

g)   Zhong Qi (Central Qi): Qi of the Stomach and Spleen, which are part of the Middle Heater.

h)   Zheng Qi (Correct Qi): generic term for the types of Qi whose function is to protect the body from invasion by external pathogenic factors.

The diseases of Qi are:

I.   Poor Qi: usually due to overwork

or irregular diet. The Qi most prone to this alteration is that of the Spleen (anorexia), Lung

(dyspnea), Heart (palpitations) or Kidney (asthma, polaciuria);

II.   Submerged Qi: submersion causing organs to prolapse. Usually occurs with the Spleen and Kidney Qi.

III.   Stagnant Qi: failure to move which occurs mainly with the Liver, Intestines and Lungs;

IV. Qi rebellion: occurs when Qi flows in the wrong direction, usually with the

Stomach and Spleen.

XEN

It is a very dense form of Qi, called Blood. The Gu Qi produced by the Spleen is sent to the Lungs and, through the action of Zong Qi, is propelled to the Heart, where it is transformed into Xen, with the help of Yuan Qi. Another organ that influences the formation of Xen is the Kidney. It stores Jing, which produces Marrow. Bone marrow contributes to the formation of Xen. It can be said that Xen is generated from the interaction of post-celestial Qi (Spleen and Stomach - Gu Qi) with pre-celestial Qi (Kidney). Its function is to nourish the body, moisten the bodily tissues and house the mind.

In relation to the organs, Xen has the following relationship with them: the Heart governs Xen and the blood vessels; the Spleen originates Xen; the Liver stores Xen; the Lung helps the Spleen send Gu Qi to the Heart and controls the blood channels and vessels; the Kidney has Yuan Qi which helps form blood and the Kidney Essence which can also be transformed into Xen.

Xen's diseases are:

I.   Deficiency: usually caused by a deficiency of

Spleen Qi and Stomach Qi;

II.   Heat: often occurs due to heat in the liver;

III.   Stasis: failure to move can be caused by the stagnation of Qi in the liver due to either heat or cold.

JING

Jing represents "Essence", something derived from the refinement of a harder substance, which needs to be guarded and cared for. There are three different types of essence, which have the following functions: growth, reproduction and development; being the basis of Kidney Qi; producing Marrow; being the basis of constitutional strength; being the basis of the Three Treasures (Jing-Qi-

Shen).

a) Pre-celestial essence: represents the combination of energies at conception, an energy that nourishes the embryo and fetus during pregnancy. It depends on the nourishment derived from the mother's Kidney, giving strength and vitality to the new being formed. It has a direct link to the Fire of the Gate of Life (Ming Men). After birth, the pre-Celestial Essence is transformed into the Kidney Essence until puberty.

b) Post-Celestial Essence: is extracted from the food and fluids of the Stomach and Spleen after birth. When the Post-Celestial Essence unites with the Air coming from the lungs, Qi is formed.

c) Kidney Essence: derived from the pre-Celestial and post-Celestial Essence, it is hereditary and determines the individual's constitution. It interacts with the post-Celestial Essence and is replenished by it. It remains stored in the Kidney and circulates in the body through the Eight Extraordinary Vessels. It makes an important contribution to growth, development, sexual maturation, reproduction, conception, pregnancy, menopause and ageing.

Regarding the functions of Essence:

1. Growth, reproduction and development: In children, it controls the growth of bones, teeth, hair, normal brain development and sexual maturity. After puberty, reproductive function and fertility. It is essential for successful conception and pregnancy. It is directly related to ageing. In men, it has a cycle of 8 years and in women 7 years.

2. Essence as the basis of Kidney Qi: Promotes interaction between Kidney Essence, Kidney Yin, Kidney Qi and Kidney Yang. Kidney Essence is the basis of Kidney Yin to produce Kidney Qi through the action of Kidney Yang.

3. Essence produces Marrow: The Marrow produced by the essence generates the bone marrow, the spinal cord and the brain.

4. Essence as the basis of constitutional strength: Essence is one of the

factors responsible for constitutional strength, which defends against pathogenic factors, along with Defensive Qi.

5.   Essence as the basis of the San Bao - Three Treasures (Jing- Qi-Shen): Essence, Qi and Mind are the fundamental physical and psychic substances of the human being. Essence represents the state of condensation of the densest and hardest Qi, Qi is more rarefied and Shen is the most subtle and material.

This combination is represented by the three organs: Xin, Wei/Pi and Shen.

JIN YE

Bodily fluids originate from food and liquids, which are transformed and separated by the Spleen. The fluid portion, considered pure, goes up to the lung, some of which is dispersed through the skin and some goes to the kidney. The so-called impure portion goes up to the Small Intestine, where it is separated into a pure portion that goes to the Bladder and an impure portion that goes down to the Large Intestine. In the Bladder, the pure fluids rise, turning into sweat. The impure ones flow downwards and become urine.

Há two types of bodily fluids:

a)   Jin: these are clear, pure, watery fluids that circulate with the Wei Qi on the outside. Their function is to moisten and nourish. They are represented by sweat, tears, saliva and mucus. It is also a component of the fluid part of Xen.

b)   Ye: these are turbid, heavy and dense fluids that circulate with the Ying Qi inside. Their function is to moisten joints, the spinal cord, the brain and the bone marrow.

Qi produces the Bodily Fluids, maintains them, transforms them and also transports them. Xen nourishes and supplies Jun Ye while Jin Ye constantly supplies Xue and transforms it into a finer fluid.

Jin Ye's illnesses are:

I.   Deficiency: dryness;

II.   Accumulation: edema, humidity or phlegm

SHEN

It is the most immaterial and subtle type of Qi. It originates from the prenatal Essences of the mother and father. After birth, the Essence is stored in the Kidney and then the Mind of the being is formed. This is housed in the Heart.

The functions of the Mind are: consciousness, thought, memory, insight, cognition, sleep, intelligence, wisdom, ideas, affections, feelings and senses.

Shen's diseases:

I.   Overshadowed or emptied mind: causes loss of consciousness;

II.   Weak or deficient mind: oligophrenia, slow and numb thinking, also affecting memory;

III.   Phlegm-clogged, degenerated mind: causes mental illness, psychosis;

IV.   A restless, troubled mind: it disturbs sleep;

V.   Mind affected by intense emotions: anger (Liver), sadness (Lung), worry (Spleen), fear (Kidney)

VI.   Mind affected by altered senses: smell (Lung), taste (Spleen), hearing (Kidney), sight (Liver)

3. Zang Fu Theory

The Zang Fu are the organs and viscera of the body. They are classified into three groups: a) six Zang; b) six Fu and c) extraordinary Fu.

a)   Zang: their characteristic is to produce and preserve vital substances, they are Yin. They connect with the bodily orifices.

1.   Pi (spleen-pancreas): manifests in the lips, nourishes the muscles, externalizes in the mouth. It is related to thought. Its fluid is serous saliva and its feeling is worry. It transforms water and food through digestion, absorbs, transports and distributes them throughout the body, moistening and nourishing the tissues. Ascends the essence of food. Keeps Xue circulating in the vessels.

When in disharmony, it manifests itself with: edema, loss of appetite, fatigue, dizziness, flatulence, diarrhea, prolapses, hematochezia, hematuria and metrorrhagia.

2.   Fei (lung): manifests itself in the hair, moistens and strengthens the skin and externalizes itself in the nose. It is related to the corporeal soul (Po). Its fluid is nasal mucus and its feeling is sadness and melancholy, which can consume the body's Qi when they persist. It is in charge of the functioning of Qi and breathing. It disperses Qi, Jing and Jin Ye throughout the body. Disseminates Wei Qi by controlling the opening and closing of skin pores. Descends Qi from Fei to keep the respiratory tract clean. It clears and regulates the passage of water. Coordinates visceral activities.

When out of harmony, it manifests as: dyspnea, a feeling of pressure on the chest, coughing, asthma, nasal obstruction, runny nose, sneezing, itchy throat, hoarseness, dysphonia, anhidrosis, excess mucus or nasal dryness.

3.   Shen (kidney): externalizes in the hair, determines the condition of the bones and bone marrow, externalizes in the ears, urethra, genitalia and anus. It is related to the will. Its fluid is thick saliva and its feeling is fear and fright. It

stores the Jing. It is in charge of development and reproduction through the Qi of Shen (Yang), which originates from the Jing of Shen (Yin). The Qi of Shen contains both the Yin and Yang components of Shen, Shen being the home of water and fire. At puberty, when Shen's Qi is at its highest, it produces Tian Gui, which in turn stimulates the development of sperm in boys and menstrual discharge in girls. It regulates the metabolism of water, controlling its retention, diffusion and elimination. It controls and promotes inhalation, while Fei promotes harmonious exhalation.

Nan Jing's theory is that the right kidney is the Gate of Life (Ming Men) and the left kidney is Shen. According to Yu Tuan, both kidneys are the Ming Men.

Zhao Xianke and Sun Yi Kui state that the Ming Men reside between the two kidneys. It should be noted that the symptoms associated with Ming Men fire deficiency are similar to those of Shen Yang deficiency.

When out of harmony, it manifests as: sterility, hair loss, weak teeth, weak bones, slow development in children, urination disorders (frequent urination, enuresis, oliguria and anuria), cold back and knees, tinnitus, deafness.

4.   Gan (liver): externalizes in the nails, nourishes the tendons, externalizes in the eyes. It is related to mood. Its fluid is tears and its feeling is anger or rage. It drains and regulates the flow of Qi (ascending, descending, incoming and outgoing) and Xue.

It stores and regulates the amount of Xue in circulation. It has the mental function of withstanding fatigue and storing the spirit (Hun).

When in disharmony, it manifests as: altered menstrual flow, anger, malnutrition, tingling of the extremities, excessive dreaming, sleepwalking, hallucinations, irritation, dry eyes.

5.   Xin (heart): manifests on the face (color), is associated with the blood vessels and is externalized on the tongue. Its fluid is sweat and its feeling is joy. It is related to the mind and houses the mind. It controls the circulation of

Xue through the Qi of Xi.

When in disharmony, it manifests itself with: pale face, thin and weak pulse, palpitations, insomnia, excessive dreams, mental restlessness, delirium, slower reaction, weakened memory, anxiety.

6.   Xin Bao (pericardium): its physiology is closely related to Xin, it is the envelope of Xin and the collateral vessels. Its function is to protect Xin. It is the first to be affected when a pathogenic factor attacks Xin.

b) Fu: is characterized by conducting, digesting and absorbing water and food, as well as excreting waste; it is Yang.

1.   Wei (stomach): receives, digests and transforms food and water. Absorbs the Jing from food. Its function is to descend the contents

food.

When out of harmony, it forms cloudy substances, halitosis, abdominal distension, stuffiness, pain, constipation, foul-smelling eructation, nausea, vomiting and hiccups.

2.   Da Chang (large intestine): transports waste, absorbs excess water, forms feces and eliminates them. It depends on the proper functioning of Wei and Fei in descent and the proper regularization of metabolism by Shen.

When out of harmony, it can lead to dysentery or difficulty defecating.

3.   Pang Guang (bladder): stores and excretes urine. When out of harmony, it causes dysuria, urinary retention, frequent urination and urinary incontinence.

4.   Dan (gallbladder): stores and excretes bile. Related to courage and decisiveness.

When Gan is in disharmony, the excretion of bile is affected, generating distension in the hypochondrium, inappetence, abdominal distension and pasty stools.

5.   Xiao Chang (small intestine): receives, transforms and absorbs food. It

separates the clear (Jing) from the turbid (waste sent to Da Chang, turbid water sent to Pang Guang).

When out of harmony, this leads to abnormalities in digestion and absorption, altered urination and defecation.

6. San Jiao (triple heater): controls the activities of Qi in the body (ascending, descending, entering and leaving). It is responsible for the path through which water and body fluids are transported.

Upper Jiao (Shang Jiao): located above the diaphragm, it houses Xin and Fei and contains the head and face. It raises and disperses Qi.

Middle Jiao (Zhong Jiao): between the diaphragm and the navel. It is the pivot of ascending and descending. Source of Qi and Xue production and encompasses the functions of Wei and Pi.

Lower Jiao (Xia Jiao): located below the navel. It houses Xiao Chang, Da Chang, Shen and Pang Guang. Contains Jing and Xue stored in the Shen and Gan and the Yuan Qi of the Ming Men. It excretes waste and urine.

When out of harmony, this manifests as difficulty in urinating and oedema due to fluid retention.

c) Extraordinary Fu: they are airtight, do not come into direct contact with water and food, and have the function of preserving vital substances. They store Jing Yin and the resources necessary for the growth and movement of the human body. They don't have related internal-external organs and are not classified as Yin or Yang.

1. Brain: the medulla concentrates to form the brain. It controls mental activity and thought. Many of the brain's functions are attributed to the Zang: Xin houses the mind and ensures pleasure; Fei stores Po (corporeal soul) and is related to sorrow; Pi houses thought and aids thinking; Gan stores Hun (spirit) and can be related to anger; Shen stores willpower and is related to fear.

The disharmonies are: Xin obscured by mucus, Xin attacked by mucus-fire, pathogenic heat attacking Xin Bao, disharmony of coordination between Xin and Shen, Gan Qi stagnation, Gan fire rising, Gan internal wind agitation, Shen Jing deficiency.

2.   Marrow: the Jing can be transformed into marrow. It relates to the body's physical strength and mental balance.

When insufficient, it leads to lassitude, hearing and speech abnormalities.

3.   Bones: when Shen's Jing is sufficient, the bone marrow is well nourished and forms strong, solid bones, which are important for the structure of the human body.

4.   Blood vessels: Pi controls the flow of Xue within the blood vessels. The vessels carry Xue to be distributed to all organs and tissues.

5.   Biliary vesicle: this is also an extraordinary fu because it stores the essence, as well as excreting and storing bile.

6.   Uterus: produces menstrual flow and is responsible for pregnancy, protecting and supporting the fetus. But the production and regulation of menstruation are controlled by the Chong Mai and Ren Mai.

The Zang Fu must be in balance and coordinated, otherwise they can manifest disorders or illnesses. Many illnesses are thought to start in the Fu and, if they persist, move on to the Zang. Diseases involving the Fu are generally syndromes of excess and those involving the Zang, of deficiency.

There is a connection between the Zang Fu to form an inner-outer relationship: Pi and Wei, Fei and Da Chang, Shen and Pang Guang, Gan and Dan, Xin and Xiao Chang, Xin Bao and San Jiao.

4. Theory of the Five Elements

The five elements are the essential constituents of nature. There is an interdependence and interrestriction that keeps them connected and moving. All the phenomena of the tissues, organs, physiology and pathology of the human body are explained by this theory.

Each element represents characteristics of nature and the human body. They are:

a) Wood:
Direction: east
Season: spring
Climate: wind
Color: green
Taste: sour
Organ: liver

Viscera: gallbladder
"Organ": eyes
Tissue: tendon
Emotion: angry
Sound: scream

b) Fire:
Direction: south
Season: summer
Climate: heat
Color: red
Taste: bitter
Organ: heart

Viscera: intestine slender
"Organ": tongue
Tissue: vascular
Emotion: joy
Sound: laughter

c) Earth:
Direction: center
Season: start/end of summer
Climate: humid
Color: yellow
Emotion: thought

Taste: sweet
Organ: spleen-pancreas
Viscera: stomach
"Organ": mouth
Tissue: muscle
Sound: singing

d) Metal:
Direction: west
Season: fall
Climate: dry
Color: white
Taste: spicy
Organ: lung

Viscera: intestine thick
"Organ": nose
Tissue: skin and hair
Emotion: concern
Sound: crying

e) Water:
Direction: north
Season: winter
Climate: cold

Viscera: bladder
"Organ": ear
Tissue: bone

Color: black   Emotion: fear
Taste: salty   Sound: moaning
Organ: kidney

Among the five elements, there is the relationship of inhibition and generation. When the term generation is used, it has the idea of producing, growing, promoting. Thus, wood generates fire, fire generates earth, earth generates metal, metal generates water, water generates wood.

The wood burns and turns to ash, which is incorporated into the earth. Under great pressure, the earth produces metals. From metals and rocks come water sources. Water gives life to plants, generating wood, and so the cycle of nature closes. This relationship of generation is called the mother-child relationship, where the generating element is the mother and the generated element is the child.

On the other hand, there is the relationship of inhibition, which is the so-called grandparent-grandchild relationship, in which there is the idea of combat, restriction and control. Inhibition occurs in the following sequence: wood inhibits earth, earth inhibits water, water inhibits fire, fire inhibits metal and metal inhibits wood. This means that metal can cut wood. Rocks and metals in the soil prevent the growth of trees representing wood. The wood grows and absorbs nutrients from the soil, impoverishing it. The roots of trees, when too long, pierce and crack the earth. The earth prevents water from spreading by absorbing it. Water extinguishes fire and fire melts metal.

There is also counter-inhibition, when the element is abundant and inhibits in the opposite direction. Generally, water inhibits fire, but if fire is in abundance and water is in short supply, water is inhibited by fire.

Applying the theory of the five elements

Each organ and viscera is represented by one of the five elements. When one of them is weakened, it generates signs and symptoms corresponding to diseases. And for their treatment we can use the theory of the five elements, with the relationships of generation and inhibition and counter-inhibition.

When the heart is weakened, we must tone up its mother, the liver. If the heart is overactive, we have to reduce its energy through its child: the spleen-pancreas. This explanation can also be understood in Western medicine. The liver supplies the body with glucose, a vital source of energy for the myocardium. The heart uses the energy provided by the oxygen that also comes from the lungs. The lung also needs the energy of the glucose generated by the liver to carry out its functions. And part of the blood volume comes from the spleen-pancreas to the liver. In this way, an imbalance in one organ can have its cause in another. And disease can cause imbalances in other systems.

5. Free Theme

ACUPUNCTURE IN THE TREATMENT OF PATIENTS WITH CHRONIC LOW BACK PAIN AT UBS LUTHER KING IN FRANCISCO BELTRÀO: CASE REPORTS

Vinicius Urbanowiski Ramos[1]

Joana Perotta Titon[2]

SUMMARY

Chronic pain is characterized as continuous or recurring pain that persists for at least three months and which generally does not respond adequately to conventional medical treatments. Chronic pain in the lumbar region has reached epidemic levels in Brazil and is highly disabling, but the application of acupuncture in these cases has shown interesting results, with pain reduction and functional improvement at low cost. The aim of this study is to report the effects of acupuncture, complementary to conventional treatment, in four patients with chronic low back pain treated in the public health system. A descriptive statistical analysis was carried out of the results of the McGill-Br pain questionnaires and the visual analogue scale (VAS) present in the medical records of patients who took part in the Pain Group in April and May 2017, at the UBS in the Luther King neighborhood of Francisco Beltrâo. After the intervention period, according to the evaluation of the parameters intensity, temporal pattern, pain index and use of analgesic medication, described in the medical records, there was a significant improvement in all patients. The pain reported went from frequent to more sporadic; the pain index decreased in the sensory, affective, subjective and mixed groups; the average VAS pain score varied from 6.25 to 3.25; two patients discontinued the use of analgesic medication, one started using drugs with less analgesic potency and the fourth

[1] Medical student at the State University of Western Paranà - UNIOESTE Campus of Francisco Beltrâo, in 2017, e-mail: vinicius.ramos2@unioeste.br.
[2] Professor supervising the article presented as a requirement for the degree in Medicine, email: joanaperotta@gmail.com.

changed the frequency of medication use from daily to weekly after the sessions. The responses obtained by patients with chronic low back pain described in this report indicate that the use of acupuncture for individuals with the same problem could be interesting, due to the cost-benefit ratio and the absence of reported side effects. The responses obtained by patients with chronic low back pain described in this report indicate that the use of this treatment modality could be interesting for improving pain.

Keywords: Acupuncture. Low back pain. Chronic pain.

INTRODUCTION

Chronic pain can be characterized as continuous or recurrent pain lasting at least three months, persistent beyond the expected period considering its etiology and refractory to conventional medical treatments (MERSKEY, 1994). Unlike acute pain, which is related to the body's integrity defense mechanisms, chronic pain not only represents a symptom, but is also associated with a dysfunction of the somatosensory system, which persists beyond the resolution of the etiological process (TEIXEIRA, 2009). It is usually accompanied by symptoms such as dysesthesia, hyperalgesia and allodynia. Because it is debilitating, long-lasting and often does not respond to conventional methods of analgesia, chronic pain represents suffering, progressive disability and poor quality of life for the patient, as well as high direct and indirect costs for the health system (GRÜNENTHAL, 2014).

Pain in the lumbar region has reached epidemic levels in the general population. In Brazil, around 10 million people are incapacitated by this condition and 70% of the population will experience at least one episode of low back pain in their lifetime. In 7 to 10% of this group, the symptoms persist for more than six months. The conventional treatments available have proved to be of little or no use in relieving chronic low back pain (SILVA, FASSA E VALE, 2004).

Chronic low back pain has various causes in its development, from neurological and biomechanical alterations in the case of neuromusculoskeletal disorders to psychological aspects (TEIXEIRA, 1999). As a result, the search for a broader therapy that covers the various aspects of this type of pain has begun (TOBO, 2010).

Acupuncture has been used as a therapy for various painful conditions (STIVAL, 2014). This Chinese medicinal technique, which consists of inserting needles into specific points on the body, has been used for over 4,000 years to relieve pain and treat illnesses, and its effect has been demonstrated in various situations for the treatment of chronic musculoskeletal pain (MENEZES, 2010). There are no definitive studies proving the histological or electromagnetic characteristics of acupuncture points, however the topographical description of such points usually corresponds to locations on the vasculonervous axes adjacent to them (PLUMER, 1980).

When applied to patients suffering from chronic low back pain, acupuncture showed clinically relevant short-term benefits in pain reduction and functional improvement, when compared to no treatment and when associated with conventional medical treatment (LIU et al, 2015).

Several studies have sought to understand the physiological response caused by acupuncture. Changes in brain electrical activity and in the thalamus, a structure that participates in the neuromodulation of pain, are physiological changes produced in the human body by acupuncture (MENEZES, 2010). The first scientific evidence that the analgesia obtained after using this method depends on a humoral mechanism was published by the Research Group of Acupuncture Anaesthesia in 1974. In this experiment, acupuncture caused analgesia in a rabbit, which then had its CSF (cerebrospinal fluid) removed and used to replace the CSF of a second rabbit, not treated with acupuncture, which began to show the effect of analgesia, thus demonstrating that the anesthesia caused by acupuncture is mediated by central neurotransmitter substances (LUNDEBERG, 2001). This relationship was later observed in humans, with an increase in endogenous opioid peptides in the plasma or cerebrospinal fluid of individuals undergoing electroacupuncture (SJOLUND, 1977).

Numerous studies have demonstrated neural interaction in the process of conducting painful stimuli. The mechanism of acupuncture can be explained in a more didactic way when separated into three levels of action: peripheral, segmental and supra-segmental:

A) Peripheral: A-delta fiber receptors are stimulated with the insertion of the needle, and this is fundamental for the cascade of segmental and supra-segmental responses. The application of the needle generates controlled local inflammation, causing the release of neuropeptides. In addition, peripheral nitric oxide is released, inducing local vasodilation and relieving the pain resulting from ischemia, as well as reducing tumor necrosis factor (TNF) and other pro-inflammatory substances, which cause the onset and maintenance of local inflammatory signs.

B) Segmental: acupuncture also affects muscle spindles by triggering sensory afferent fibers whose stimuli, when conducted to the medulla, reflexively activate myorelaxing effectors, resulting in distension of the corresponding tendons. In addition, the response of sympathetic fibers after injury is an additional cause of the production of pro-inflammatory mediators in the peripheral sensory endings. This stimulus, over prolonged periods, causes plastic changes in the spinal cord, which intensify the painful sensation. The neuromodulatory action of acupuncture then acts to control pain through the segmental autonomic nervous system.

C) Supra-segmental: the peripheral stimulation of acupuncture reaches the gray matter of the midbrain, *locus ceruleus*, paragigantocellular and dorsal reticular subnuclei in the medulla. All these connections occur from the stimulation of the A-delta fibers by acupuncture and are intended to inhibit the progression of nociceptive information from the C fibers (RONDINELLI, 2009).

Needling at specific points during an acupuncture session therefore activates opioid and non-opioid pathways, which are responsible for modulating pain. The consequence of this activation is the release of certain substances in the brain such as endorphins, which belong to a subtype of neuropeptide called opioid, known for its anesthetic properties (MENEZES, 2010).

Serotoninergic pathways are also implicated in the origin of acupuncture-induced analgesia, since an increase in serotonin concentration was observed in the CSF and in the neuronal structures of the lower brainstem in guinea pigs after application of this technique. Furthermore, the use of serotonergic blockers was found to interrupt the action of acupuncture, confirming that opioid pathways are not solely responsible for the analgesic effect of acupuncture (MENEZES, 2010).

Recent guidelines from the American College of Physicians (ACP) strongly recommend that, when treating chronic low back pain, patients and doctors initially choose non-pharmacological therapeutic resources, including acupuncture. This type of intervention is indicated as a first-line option in the treatment of this condition, as it is associated with less harm to the patient when compared to pharmacological options in general (QASEEM et al., 2017).

Bearing these aspects in mind, it is also interesting to consider the cost-benefit ratio of using acupuncture.

According to the document "WHO Traditional Medicine - Definitions", published by the WHO in 2002, acupuncture should be encouraged by its member countries for various reasons, such as its low cost and high effectiveness (Santos, SANTOS et al, 2009). Since the cost of this therapeutic method is low, its provision by the public health system can help to reduce the high costs of outpatient services maintained by the government, which include spending on medicines, exams and the involvement of numerous specialists in dealing with a single patient (GÓIS, 2007).

In addition to this positive stimulus in the cost-benefit ratio, other benefits have been noted in studies such as increased range of motion, improved quality of life and psychological perception of pain (GODOY et al, 2014).

Therefore, due to the effects it has on neurotransmitters associated with pain and depression, acupuncture is accepted as an appropriate therapeutic modality for relieving chronic pain (STIVAL, 2014).

Based on a sample of selected medical records, this study aims to assess whether there has been a significant effect on pain reduction in patients with chronic low back pain undergoing acupuncture treatment at a Basic Health Unit in the municipality of Francisco Beltrao - PR.

MATERIALS AND METHODS

Due to the high number of people who suffer from various chronic pains and seek relief from them in public health services, the health team at UBS Luther King selected patients with chronic low back pain to join the so-called "Pain Group". The patients included in the group, who were already using drug treatment, then began to associate it with weekly acupuncture sessions, with the systematic recording of clinical data being carried out by the professionals responsible in each patient's medical records.

A descriptive study was carried out, reviewing the medical records of patients who took part in the Pain Group in April and May 2017, at the UBS in the Luther King neighborhood of Francisco Beltrâo.

In order to assess the response to acupuncture treatment, a descriptive statistical analysis was carried out on the results of the pain grading instruments in the medical records, comparing the results before and after the sessions.

The location of the needles was chosen according to the patient's complaints. They were inserted into the selected points, respecting the anatomical location described by Traditional Chinese Medicine. The procedures were carried out by a medical professional qualified to apply the treatment, which consisted of weekly acupuncture sessions for eight weeks.

The patients who took part in the "Pain Group" during the period analyzed were subjected to two evaluation instruments, described below:

1- **The visual analog scale (VAS) is** a one-dimensional instrument used to assess pain intensity. It is a line with the ends numbered 0-10. One end of the line is marked "no pain" and the other "worst pain imaginable";

2- **McGill-Br Pain Questionnaire (MPQ)**, a multidimensional instrument that assesses various aspects of pain using words (descriptors) that the patient must choose to express their painful impression. A body diagram was added for better localization and assessment of periodicity and duration. Some examples of descriptors present in the questionnaire that help to better understand the patient's painful sensation are: *sharp, stinging, cutting, torturing, tingling, squeezing, numbing, radiating, etc.*

The characteristics and pain index were assessed using the third part of the McGill-Br questionnaire, with descriptive terms distributed into four groups: a group of sensory responses to the pain experience, such as mechanical and thermal properties; a group of affective dimensions, which refer to tension and fear; a group of descriptors evaluating the overall pain experience; and a mixed group. Within each group, each term marked by the patient corresponds to a value, which was added up to form the pain index before and after the intervention.

The virtual analog pain scale was applied immediately before and after each session and the McGill Pain Questionnaire (MPQ) before the first and after the last session of acupuncture treatment.

RESULTS AND DISCUSSION

Initially, seven patients were selected to take part in the Pain Group, but three could not be included in the report: two because they had not filled in the questionnaires correctly, which meant that the information in the medical records was incomplete and could not be analyzed, and the third because he did not attend the eight acupuncture sessions, claiming personal reasons. Therefore, four medical records contained sufficient information for the report.

All the records belonged to female patients, aged between 44 and 78, with an average age of 59.75. The sites of pain reported by the study group were: lumbar, cervical, posterior thigh and foot. They all had low back pain in common, with three patients having deep, diffuse low back pain and one patient having deep, localized low back pain, according to the first part of the McGill-Br questionnaire.

Analyzing the parameters pain index, temporal pattern, intensity and use of analgesic medication, it was possible to observe that there was a significant improvement in pain in all patients after the intervention period.

The sum of the values assigned to each descriptive term on the McGill-Br Questionnaire constitutes the pain index before and after acupuncture treatment. The descriptors selected by the patients fall into four groups: sensory, affective, subjective evaluation and mixed. The comparison of these values showed that there was a reduction in the average index in all the groups mentioned, as shown in Figure 1. It can be seen that, before treatment, most of the terms mentioned by the patients were part of the sensory group (mechanical and thermal perceptions),

making up the highest index before and which, perhaps as a consequence, showed the greatest variation in numerical values when compared to the post-acupuncture value.

FIGURE 1 - Comparison of the mean pain index in the groups before and after the intervention period, using the McGILL-Br questionnaire.

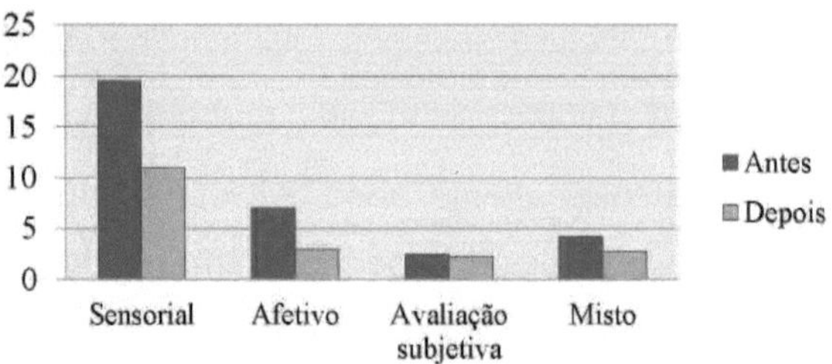

Source: Records of patients in the pain group at UBS Luther King, 2017.

In addition, the McGill-Br questionnaire uses a scale to assess the temporal pattern of pain made up of words graded from 1 to 3, where 1 represents continuous, stable, constant pain; 2 represents rhythmic, periodic, intermittent pain; and 3 represents brief, momentary, transient pain. All the patients experienced an improvement in the temporal pattern of pain, going from more frequent pain to more sporadic pain, as shown in Table 1.

TABLE 1. Temporal pattern of pain before and after acupuncture treatment.

Patient	Before the intervention	After intervention
Patient 1	1	2
Patient 2	1	3
Patient 3	2	3
Patient 4	1	2

Source: Records of patients in the pain group at UBS Luther King, 2017.

All the patients showed an improvement in the visual analog pain scale (VAS) after the proposed intervention, with the average of the 4 patients before the first session being 6.25 (classified as moderate to severe) and the average after the last session being 3.25 (mild to moderate), as shown in Table 2.

Table 2. Variation in the numerical pain intensity scale before and after intervention.

Patient	Before the intervention	After intervention
Patient 1	8	5

Patient 2	4	0
Patient 3	8	5
Patient 4	5	3

Source: Records of patients in the pain group at UBS Luther King, 2017.

The change in the pharmacological treatments used by the patients before and after the acupuncture intervention also showed a reduction in the intensity of the pain in the cases under study. After the eight sessions, two patients reported that they had stopped using any medication for analgesia, one started to use drugs with less analgesic potency, falling into the "mild pain" category of the analgesic ladder and only one did not change the medication used, but reported a change in the frequency of use, from daily to weekly, because she noticed a greater persistence of the relief obtained with the ingestion of the medication. Table 1 summarizes the treatment variations and details the drugs used by each patient.

Several studies looking at acupuncture in the treatment of chronic low back pain have generally shown positive results, suggesting that the treatment is effective in improving patients' quality of life.

In all four cases under study, the patients were female. This factor may have influenced the positive responses obtained in pain control after treatment, as indicated by an experiment involving 11378 patients with chronic low back pain, in which pain reduction was significantly more pronounced among women (WITT, 2006). According to the same study, other variables such as education, age and physical and mental quality of life also seem to have an influence on the response to treatment, but this information was not available in the medical records used.

Table 1. Pharmacological treatment used by each patient before and after the acupuncture sessions.

Patient	Drug treatment prior to acupuncture	Drug treatment

	sessions	acupuncture post-sessions
Patient 1	Nonsteroidal anti-inflammatory drug associated with opioid for constant use	Analgesic (paracetamol) for occasional use
Patient 2	Anti-inflammatory (nimesulide) and analgesic (paracetamol) for weekly use	None
Patient 3	Muscle relaxant, corticosteroid and analgesic	None
Patient 4	Anti-inflammatory drugs (torsilax and nimesulide) and tricyclic antidepressants (amitriptyline)	Analgesic (paracetamol), anti-inflammatory (nimesulide) and tricyclic antidepressant (amitriptyline)

Source: Records of patients in the pain group at UBS Luther King, 2017.

HAAKE et al. (2007) showed an improvement in all the clinical parameters assessed in patients who received acupuncture treatment and also in patients who underwent only needling at non-acupuncture points, when compared to the control group who received only conventional treatment. Among the parameters assessed, one that decreased significantly when compared to the control group was the use of analgesic medication, as occurred in three of the cases reported here.

In a multicenter, randomized, controlled study, Cherkin et al. evaluated the effectiveness of acupuncture in the treatment of chronic low back pain. In total, 638 patients included in the study were divided into 4 groups: treatment with individualized acupuncture; treatment with standardized acupuncture, minimal intervention with superficial needling (acupuncture simulation); and conventional treatment (control group). The study showed a curious result: there was a significant difference when comparing the response of the control group to the response of the other groups, which received some form of acupuncture. Among these, the difference was not significant, although the improvement in pain was slightly greater in the group that received standardized acupuncture (CHERKIN, 2009).

The fact that the placebo effect of simulated acupuncture was perceived in the studies cited could cast doubt on the results obtained in the cases reported here. It is not possible to say with certainty whether the effects of the treatment were physiological (specific) or psychological (unspecific), reflecting the patients' positive expectations of acupuncture when compared to conventional medicine; the more intensive contact with the medical professional and the experience of an invasive technique such as needling. In any case, even if the effects were psychological, they promoted a better quality of life and a sense of well-being for the patients.

Lam and colleagues came to different conclusions about the placebo effect attributed to simple needling. They identified 25 randomized controlled trials comparing real acupuncture with sham acupuncture and other treatments to evaluate the therapy of chronic pain and chronic low back pain. The analysis of these studies led to the conclusion that acupuncture relieves chronic low back pain and that it is more effective in producing analgesia than simulated acupuncture. However, they point out that the data must be interpreted in the context of the limitations found, such as the heterogeneity of the studies included in this meta-analysis and the low methodological quality of several of them (LAM et al, 2013).

Because it has recently shown similar responses to those presented by Lam, acupuncture continues to be recommended by the American College of Physicians, which evaluated randomized controlled trials and systematic reviews in publications from 2015 and 2016. The recent conclusion was that this technique has a moderate effect on reducing chronic pain and improving lumbar function compared to the effects in the group without acupuncture, and a moderate effect on pain, with no noticeable effect on lumbar function compared to simulated acupuncture (QASEEM et al., 2017).

Neurosciences consider acupuncture to be a medical procedure of peripheral neuromodulation, through physical stimulation, which combines tradition and modernity and presupposes a systemic, interdisciplinary and interprofessional approach, always aiming to alleviate pain and suffering (RONDINELLI, 2009). The positive results presented in this report indicate that the use of this ancient technique, associated or not with pharmacological treatment, is interesting as an initial alternative for patients with chronic low back pain or those with an inadequate response to the restricted use of medication.

FINAL CONSIDERATIONS

In the evolution of the four cases reported at UBS Luther King in Francisco Beltrâo, acupuncture, in addition to routine care, resulted in clinically relevant benefits for patients with chronic low back pain. There is no report of another primary health care unit in the municipality offering acupuncture as a treatment option for these patients. The responses obtained by patients with chronic low back pain described in this report may indicate that the use of this treatment modality for individuals with the same problem in other public healthcare units could be interesting, due to the cost-benefit ratio and the absence of reported side effects.

More studies are needed to confirm this hypothesis, since the absence of a group of patients receiving placebo needling could raise the question of whether the psychological effect (non-specific) prevailed over the physiological effect (specific). What's more, other non-specific effects may have contributed to the good therapeutic response, such as low expectations of conventional medicine, greater contact with the doctor and experience of an invasive treatment technique.

Considering the potential for pain relief that acupuncture has demonstrated, the effects of using this technique in patients with chronic low back pain who have already been using conventional treatments, but without an adequate response, is still a field that can be widely studied.

6. Bibliographical references:

CHERKIN, D. C., et al. A randomized trial comparing acupuncture, simulated acupuncture, and usual care for chronic low back pain. **Archives of Internal Medicine,** v. 169 n. 9, p. 858-66, 2009.

CHRIST, C. D. Monograph: Acupuncture and chronic pain. **Revista dor, pesquisa, clinica e terapèutica.** v. 7, n. 1, jan/feb/mar. 2006.

DELLAROZA, M. S. G. et al. Characterization of chronic pain and analgesic methods used by elderly people in the community. **Revista Associaçao Mèdica Brasileira**, v. 54, p.36-41, 2008.

GODOY, J. R. P.; NERY, W., THEOPHILO, E. Effect of acupuncture on low back pain: literature review. **Universitas: Ciências da saùde**, Brasilia. v.12, n. 1, p.49-57. 2014.

GÓIS, A. L. B. Acupuncture, multidisciplinary specialty: an option in public services applied to the elderly. **Revista Brasileira de Geriatria Gerontologia**, v.10(1), p. 87-100, 2007.

GUNNAR, A. Epidemiologic aspects on low-back pain in industry. **Spine,** v. 6, p. 53-60, jan. 1981.

HAAK, M. et al. German Acupuncture Trials (GERAC) for chronic low back pain: randomized, multicenter, blinded, parallel-group trial with 3 groups. Archives of Internal Medicine, v. 167, n. 17, p. 1892-8, 2007.

KAWAKITA, K.; OKADA, K. Acupuncture therapy: mechanism of action, efficacy, and safety: a potential intervention for psychogenic disorders? **Biopsychosocial Medicine.** v. 8, n. 4, p. 1-7, 2014.

LAM, M; GALVIN, R; CURRY, P. Effectiveness of acupuncuture for nonspecific chronic low back pain: a systematic review and metaanalysis. **Spine,** v. 38, n. 24, p. 2124-38, nov. 2013.

LIU, Z. et al. Acupuncture for Low Back Pain: An Overview of Systematic

Reviews. **Evidence-Based Complementary and Alternative Medicine**. v. 2015, mar. 2015.

LUNDEBERG, T. Effects of sensory stimulation (acupuncture) on the circulatory and immune systems. in: ERNEST, E., WHITE, A.

(Acupuncture, a scientific evaluation. Sâo Paulo: Manole, 2001.

MACIOCIA, G, MING S. X. **The fundamentals of Chinese medicine**. 2. Ed. Sâo Paulo: Roca, 2014.

MENEZES, C. R. O., MOREIRA, A. C. P., BRANDÂO, W. B. Neurophysiological basis for understanding chronic pain through Acupuncture. **Revista Dor**. v. 11, p. 161-168, 2010.

MERSKEY, H. **Classification of chronic pain: descriptions of chronic pain syndromes and definitions of pain terms prepared by the international association for the study of pain**. 2. ed. Seattle: IASP; 1994

PLUMER, J. P. Anatomical findings at acupuncture loci. **Journal of Traditional Chinese Medicine**. v.8, n. 1-2, p.170-180, 1980.

QASEEM, A. et al. Noninvasive Treatments for Acute, Subacute, and Chronic Low Back Pain: A Clinical Practice Guideline From the American College of Physicians. **Annals of Internal Medicine,** American College of Physicians. v. 166, p. 514-30, feb. 2017.

RONDINELLI, M. C., SAMPAIO, W. C. Acupuncture and pain. In: NETO, O. A.; COSTA, C. M. C.; SIQUEIRA, J. T. T.; TEIXEIRA, M. J. (SBED) (Org.). **Dor: Principios e Pràtica**. 1. ed. Porto Alegre: Artmed, v. 1, p. 1009-1017, 2009.

SANTOS F. A. S.; GOUVEIA G. C.; MARTELLI P. J. L. Acupuncture in the Unified Health System and the inclusion of non-medical professionals. **Revista Brasileira Fisioterapia**, Sâo Carlos. v.13, n. 4, p.330-4, 2009.

SILVA, M. C.; FASSA, A. C. G.; VALLE, N. C. J. Chronic low back pain in an adult population in southern Brazil: prevalence and associated factors.

Caderno de Saùde Pùblica, Rio de Janeiro, v. 20, p. 377-385, Mar. 2014.

SJOLUND, B.; TERENIUS, L.; ERICSSON M. Increased cerebrospinal fluid levels of endorphins after electro-acupuncture. **Acta Physiologica Scandinavica**. v. 100, p. 382-84, 1977.

STIVAL, R. S. M. et al. Acupuncture in fibromyalgia: a randomized-controlled trial addressing immediate pain response.

Revista brasileira de reumatologia, Elsevier, v.54, p.431-436, Sep. 2014.

TEIXEIRA, M. J. Physiopathology of pain. In: NETO, O. A.; COSTA, C. M. C.; SIQUEIRA J. T. T.; TEIXEIRA, M. J. (SBED) (Org.). **Pain: Principles and Practice**. 1. ed. Porto Alegre: Artmed, 2009, v. 1, p. 145176.

TEIXEIRA, M. J. Multidisciplinary treatment of patients with pain. In: Carvalho MMMJ. **Pain: a multidisciplinary study**. Sào Paulo: Summus. p. 77-85, 1999.

TOBO, A.; EL KHOURI, M.; CORDEIRO, Q. Study of the treatment of chronic low back pain using the Posture School. **Acta Fisiàtrica**. v.17, p. 112-116, jun. 2010.

Pharmacological treatment of acute and chronic pain. São Paulo: Grünenthal, 2014. 28p.

WANG, L. G.; PAI, H. J. **Contemporary Treatise on Acupuncture and Moxibustion**. São Paulo: CEIMEC, 2005

WEN, T. S. **Classical Chinese Acupuncture**. 2. ed. Sâo Paulo, Cultrix: 1985.

WITT, C. M. et al. Pragmatic randomized trial evaluating the clinical and economic effectiveness of acupuncture for chronic low back pain. **American Journal of Epidemiology**. v. 164, p. 487-96, sep. 2006.

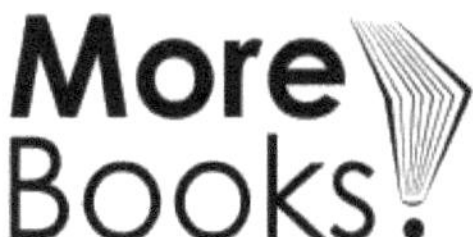

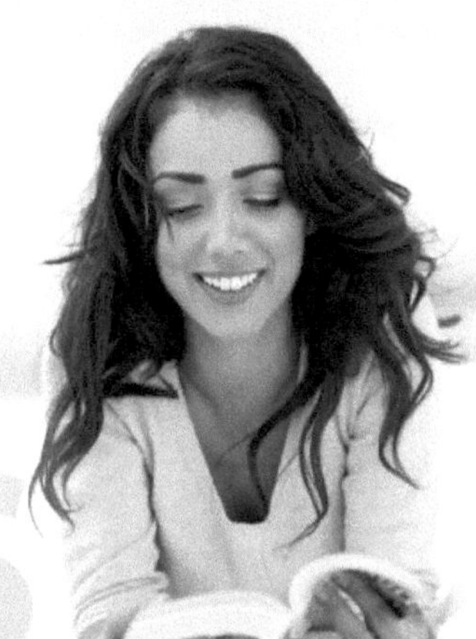

yes I want morebooks!

Buy your books fast and straightforward online - at one of world's fastest growing online book stores! Environmentally sound due to Print-on-Demand technologies.

Buy your books online at
www.morebooks.shop

Kaufen Sie Ihre Bücher schnell und unkompliziert online – auf einer der am schnellsten wachsenden Buchhandelsplattformen weltweit! Dank Print-On-Demand umwelt- und ressourcenschonend produziert.

Bücher schneller online kaufen
www.morebooks.shop

info@omniscriptum.com
www.omniscriptum.com

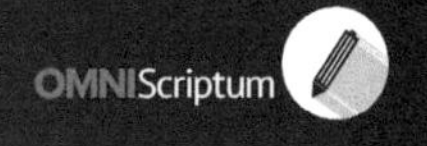

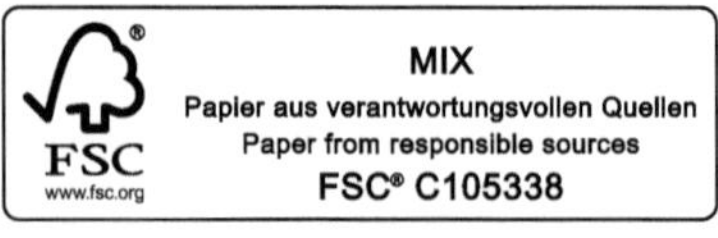

y Books on Demand GmbH, Norderstedt / Germany